CONFINED
TO THE
SIDELINES

CONFINED
TO THE
SIDELINES

New and Selected Verses

JEFF NISKER MD PhD

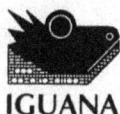

IGUANA

Publisher: Cheryl Hawley
Front cover design: Jonathan Relph

ISBN 978-1-77180-627-5 (hardcover)
ISBN 978-1-77180-626-8 (paperback)
ISBN 978-1-77180-625-1 (epub)

This is an original print edition of *Confined to the Sidelines*.

To my Mother

Contents

Introduction

Confined to the Sidelines is a juxtaposition of the poems I have written in the time of COVID with four of my related social justice poems written prior to COVID's presence. With this volume I hope to imbue new compassion in COVID-stressed health professionals, other health policy makers, and the general public, who through their votes are indeed health policy makers. We all are or will be immersed in COVID's perpetual diminishment of our health and social systems, not to mention COVID's contagious transference of aggression to humans in Canada[1] and other countries.[2]

COVID has altered many of our lives. COVID first altered mine before I ever heard the word COVID, when I developed pneumonia from COVID in February 2020, two weeks before the world learned a "virus of concern" had been rampant in Wuhan, China since autumn 2019. COVID continued to hold me in captivity after I recovered, even though I was fortunate not to become a "long hauler,"[3] as my colleagues continued to confine me to the sidelines, concerned COVID would claim me because chemotherapy had diminished my immune-response capacity to both COVID and its vaccine. This sideline confinement continues even after my third jab, and I remain banished from the hospital and my office therein, as I write and refine these verses.

I have to admit that I surreptitiously enter the hospital from time to time to exchange work with my research associate. My quiet footsteps echo loudly off the walls of the eerily silent halls; silent because all non-emergency surgeries and all non-urgency clinics have been COVID-cancelled. The Oncology Clinic next to my office cannot be cancelled, but treatment capacity is limited under some magic metric. As I walk past the Clinic's half-filled waiting room, I reminisce about the months I sat shoulder to shoulder here, consumed with collegiality for those who sat beside me, many of whom are no longer alive. The echo of my footsteps also reminisces my many happier pre-COVID years working here; happiness I hope to again experience when COVID disappears.

Until then COVID will remain the elephant in the room, even on Zoom, influencing conversations, relationships, moods, work environments, shopping-for-food environments; indeed every component of every awake hour.

Confined to the Sidelines is my only book in which my poems have remained as poems. All my other creative writings, though beginning as poems, have morphed into short stories or plays[4] for wider engagement. Several of my plays are but compilations of long prose poems interwoven into a theatre-translation format with the social justice exploration pushed forward by intermittent recitations of the actors. One of my plays, *Ruth*,[5] has only one actor who expresses a 90-minute prose poem while dramatically wheeling around the stage in her "power chair." In *Sarah's Daughters*,[6] an actor also expresses a 90-minute prose poem, this time interwoven with an on-stage performance of a cellist, who eventually becomes a second actor. In *A Child on Her Mind*,[7] six actors perform prose poems in intermittent linked sequence. For the musical play *Orchids*,[8] I wrote my poems as song lyrics, and the lauded Canadian composer Steven Hardy put music to my verses. As poetry needs no creed, nor race, nor gender, *Orchids* was last performed by an all-Black, all-woman cast in Norfolk, Virginia. As plays "have legs," my poems have been performed in six countries, as far away as Australia and South Africa, and many times in Europe, the United States, and Canada. One of my poems even morphed into the social justice novel *Patiently Waiting For....*[9]

I permitted the collection of poems in *Confined to the Sidelines* to remain as poems, as I believe the concision of poetry can be extremely helpful in healthcare education,[10] considering the tight limits of curricular minutes in health-profession schools and in national and international conference programs. Within these tight limits, poetry's precision is capable of simultaneously unpacking a topic and imbuing compassion through a tightly focused social justice lens.

To use my poems for the purpose of social justice, I eventually remove the potential distraction of end-of-line rhyme, while permitting the rhythmic lyrical sounds to engage within the margins. I acknowledge that it is the rhyme that often creates the rhythm initially to propel me in whichever direction oral sounds wish to take me. End-of-line rhyme still creeps in sometimes, as is to be expected considering the method of my poetry practice has been to dictate verses into a hand-held tape recorder, then request my generous assistant put on her stethoscope to type my intermittent heartbeats. However, as it has become increasingly difficult to find tapes, not to mention repair my aging recorder, I find myself writing verses by hand rather than attempting to disengage my brain into a new digital recorder or, perish the thought, disengage my brain from my fingers in order that verses magically appear on a computer screen.

Poetry may be making a comeback concurrent with COVID's evaporation of our classrooms, conference rooms, lecture theatres, and amphitheatres. I hope poetry's comeback continues, and poetry will be adopted widely in healthcare teaching, sharing, and thinking. I hope poetry's comeback continues, and will engage persons in all nations to make them more compassionate places for all to live in.

In the summer of 2022, I continue to be confined to the sidelines with my sunshine being the time to try to refine these verses. Poetry comes from passion and pain, from love and longing, from purpose and pleasure. Indeed, poetry comes from everything, and, equally important, poetry can contribute to everything. As COVID may be with us for many years, and poetry will be with us forever, let us employ poetry to focus an intense spotlight on the endemic problems in our health and social systems. Let us employ poetry to assist persons suffering these systems' inadequacies; inadequacies that COVID too easily laid bare at our feet.

---

1. For example, as described in Chapter VI, "COVID Aggression Condemns a Muslim Family Near Our Medical School," and in Chapter VIII, "Antivaxxer Xenophobic COVID Violence." I also observe new aggression from car and truck drivers as I run the roads that I have run for many years. Examples of this new aggression are the increased blatant blaring of car and truck horns. When I am driving I also observe the impatient aggressive cutting-in on previously calm roads.
2. As seen in the large increase in gun violence in the United States, including the murders of 19 children in Uvalde, Texas (Associated Press, "What We Know about the Uvalde, Texas, Shooting Victims"), and 10 in Buffalo, New York (Associated Press, "Mass Shooting in Buffalo, N.Y.").

3. Long haulers are persons who develop chronic illness from COVID, including "long COVID" syndrome (Siegelman, "Reflections of a COVID-19 Long Hauler"). Long-haul truckers have been in the news in 2022 for their occupation of Canada's capital Ottawa, and at border crossings, such as at Windsor, Ontario; Emerson, Manitoba; and Coutts, Alberta, in opposition to the requirements for COVID vaccination (Fraser, "Ambassador Bridge Reopens," 2022).

4. Nisker, *From Calcedonies to Orchids*, 2012.

5. See Chapter VII, "Ruth." Earlier versions of Ruth's story were published as the short story "Chalcedonies" in the *Canadian Medical Association Journal* (Nisker, 2001), and in "From the Other Side of the Fence: Stories from Health Care Professionals" (Nisker, *From the Other Side of the Fence*, 2008). I then expanded Ruth's story to a full-length play that was produced in several countries and published in my compilation *From Calcedonies to Orchids* (Nisker, 2012), as well as chapters in *Reflective Practice* (Nisker, 2010), and *Health Humanities Reader* (Nisker, 2014). I was able to honour Ruth better with the novel *Patiently Waiting For...* (Nisker, 2015).

6. Nisker, "She Lived with the Knowledge," 2004.

7. Nisker, "A Child on Her Mind," 2007.

8. Nisker, "Chalcedonies," 2001; Nisker, *From Calcedonies to Orchids*, 2012.

9. Nisker, *Patiently Waiting For...*, 2015.

10. Nisker, "She Lived with the Knowledge," 2004.

Chapter I
Confined to the COVID Sidelines

While Canada remained vaccine vacant
Airplanes lifted wealthy Canadians
Over our closed-to-car border
To Florida for vaccine
And the sunbeam vaccine would bring
To that first COVID-claustrophobic winter
Of danger to the older
And discontent to twenty-somethings[1]

The pores in our semipermeable border
Were large enough for better-off to cross
But restricted osmosis of disadvantaged
At greater risk of COVID cough
And transport through our morgues
To tractor-trailer freezers
Along with persons from long term care
And seniors not yet vaccine-protected

However four of our hospital's Execs
Dipped in the limited vaccine left
Before boarding jets for a hypocrite rest
Ignoring their own distancing requests[2]
And their blasting of nursing staff[3]
For lax cafeteria-masking
But when our Execs were dismissed
They were rewarded with enormous packages[4]

I offered to work in our COVID Clinic
But heard "We need nurses not doctors"
I offered again a month later
When our nurses requested a rest
And a large Clinic was set to open
In our region's Agriplex
But heard "We're out of vaccine
And there's none coming till late spring"

More than two years after COVID's declare
Our border no longer confines cars
But I remain confined to the COVID sidelines
Watching new variants' body counts on TV
And though I keep volunteering
To assist in our COVID Clinic
Low immunity keeps me languishing
Keeps me an impotent MD

---

1. "Winter of our discontent" from Shakespeare's *Richard III* (1594). Discontent of twenty-somethings may have participated in the hate crimes on and near our campus, including the hate crime on June 7, 2021, described in Chapter VI, "COVID Aggression Condemns a Muslim Family Near Our Medical School." This aggression was soon followed by four sexual assaults in our University's residences, and with the murder (now manslaughter) of an 18-year-old student on our campus (Dolynny, "Second Person Wanted in Connection with Western Student's Death," 2021; Dubinski, "Arrests Made after 4 Western Students Reported Sexual Assaults in Past Week," 2021).
2. Brown, "Unions Fire Back at LHSC Boss's 'Shaming' over COVID-19 Protocol Lapses," 2020.
3. Our hospital's President sent an internal email "blasting" employees for not wearing face masks, and not "physically distancing" on cafeteria and other breaks (Brown, "Unions Fire Back at LHSC Boss's 'Shaming' over COVID-19 Protocol Lapses," 2020).
4. Our hospital's President and Senior Executive Vice President received "enormous severance packages" on their dismissal after threatening to sue London Health Sciences Centre for "groundless dismissal" (Newcombe, "Sudden Departure of Two LHSC Executives Might Cost $750,000 in Severance," 2021).

Chapter II
Webinar Physicians' Cavalier Terms Promote COVID-Ventilation Triage of Disabled Persons

Webinar physicians' cavalier terms
For COVID-ventilator triage of disabled persons
Set a dangerous restriction precedent
For all persons seen as less healthy
Persons thus seen as more worthy
Of permitting death with dignity[1]
"If two MDs agree"[2] that's all you need
To be hanging judges[3] and juries

Webinar physicians' cavalier terms
Limit persons to just numbers
Entered in "clinical factor calculators"
And coloured on triage-criteria charts
Charts that set persons of difference apart
For better "return on investment"
And spread the virus of the myth
Of "finite health resources"

Webinar physicians' triage terms
Such as "we can't afford to have this"
Must be rebutted with our insist

That we can't afford not to have this
As persons are not cash to be transacted
Nor liquid assets to be liquidated
Nor currency to be based
On "predicted short-term mortality"

Webinar physicians' triage terms
Dissolve physician trust in hemlock[4]
And our profession in suspicion
Confirming the worst opinion of physicians
"If two MDs agree" with triage
We must ensure they are not one God
As physicians must not be omnipotent
Purveyors of COVID-ventilator restriction

Webinar physicians' triage terms
Spread concern that the physicians who use them
Are insensitive to persons with disabilities
And other persons of difference
For though ventilator restriction is "still hypothetical"
Hypothetical too often masks prophetical
Of the death knell of those deemed less fit[5]
Of the death knell of justice in our health system

A preliminary version of this poem was published in Impact Ethics *on May 13, 2021, yet the threat of COVID-ventilator restriction to persons with disabilities continues into 2022.*

---

1. See Chapter VII, "Ruth."
2. Quotation marks indicate exact terms used by physicians in the Webinar on COVID-ventilator restriction. Unfortunately, the Webinar did not provide the ability to cite or reference not only in healthcare journals, but the lay press. This inability makes webinars potentially dangerous in healthcare and more.
3. "A hanging judge" is the deprecating term for a judge who prefers to sentence someone to "hang by the neck until dead" rather than consider a life sentence in prison.

4. Hemlock was a common poison in ancient Greece. Prior to the ancient Greek physician Hippocrates' insistence that physicians must always act in the best interest of their patient's health, physicians were not always trusted because of their equal knowledge of poisons and medicines, and the financial reward of physicians to be assassins. If COVID promotes physicians to permit their patients to die rather than find ways to accommodate their survival by assuring access to a COVID ventilator, physicians will once again be viewed askance.
5. Hitler used the language of less fit and less human to make it easier for Germans and persons in bordering countries to accept the extermination of Jews (Dawidowicz, 1975).

Chapter III
Claustrophobia's Fear of a COVID Ventilator

Claustrophobia has been a consistent
Intimate cog of my being
Because of my recurring dream
Of trying to rescue my cousin[1]
In my dream Ronnie was ten when he had fallen
From a concrete pier into deep water
And without words disappeared down
Condemned to drown under the molten curtain

In my dream the teen me dives in
And finds him in a submerged cavern
Grasps his hand with encouragement
Begins to urgently swim him out
But I come to a fork in the tunnel
And am not sure which channel to take
And run out of breath soaked in sweat
Each night as I awake

Claustrophobia became a life sentence
When Ronnie in a non-dream drowned
Having fallen off an Institution's sleigh
Unnoticed onto a supposed-frozen lake
And while trying to walk back to Huronia[2]

Fell through a crack in the ice
With only the ears of darkness
Hearing his wordless pleas for help

Claustrophobia insists my running
Endless rungs of hospital stairs
Rather than enter an elevator
Even if the elevator is empty
And propels my feet on silent streets
And empty fields and wide trails
Finding freedom to inhale
Where open oxygen prevails

Claustrophobia excuses my refusal
To be buried in the sand
By my eager-to grandchildren
Who are confused by this refusal
And adds to the reasons I condemn discrimination
Against persons with motion restriction[3]
When physicians triage-restrict them
From intensive care ventilators[4]

Claustrophobia constricts with masking
But also with the lack of masking
Observed in emerald waves on St. Paddy's Day
And multicoloured "Frosh Week" rivers
As well as stagnant placard ponds
Perfect for hatching new variants
To prolong COVID's presence
Along with matching resentment

Claustrophobia increases with cocooning
For this fully morphed professor
Confined to the cloister of a computer screen
Engaging exclusively on Zoom
Rather than in classrooms with students

And conference rooms with colleagues
Forbidden till vaccine vanquishes
The pall of this gloom

My claustrophobia does not fear death
But fears a COVID ventilator
Against which this is an Advance Directive
To give the ventilator to another
Rather than endure claustrophobia
Which for me is worse than death
Because death comes to all of us
But claustrophobia to just some of us

---

1. I reflect further on my cousin in the short story "I'm Sorry Ronnie" (Nisker, *Love and Injustice in Medicine*, 2022).
2. Huronia was originally named "The Orillia Asylum for Idiots." Marilyn Dolmage, the sister of a man with Down Syndrome who died in Huronia from untreated pneumonia, described how those living there "had all of their citizenship rights stripped away … They were lined up to eat, they were lined up to shower" (Marlin, "A Chance for Huronia's 'Invisible' to Be Seen and Heard," 2010). Former residents of Huronia now participate in the Huronia Speakers Bureau, a speakers' series that tries "to ensure no one forgets—and people understand—the horrors they endured there" (Ballingall, "Former Huronia Residents Join Speakers' Series," 2016); other survivors of Huronia work in a research project lead by Kate Rossiter that includes a theatrical production recounting their experience at Huronia (Battersby, "Huronia Survivors Work through Their Pain," 2018).
3. I wrote of the discrimination endured by the woman I call "Ruth," with her permission, in a short story published in the *Canadian Medical Association Journal* (Nisker, "Chalcedonies," 2001), and as a full-length play produced in several countries, and published in the compendium of my plays *From Calcedonies to Orchids* (Nisker, 2012). The short story was also published in *Reflective Practice* (Nisker, 2010), and *Health Humanities Reader* (Nisker, 2014). I was able to honour "Ruth" again with my novel *Patiently Waiting For...* (Nisker, 2015), and most recently in Chapter 17 of *Love and Injustice in Medicine* (Nisker, 2022).
4. See Chapter II, "Webinar Physicians' Cavalier Terms Promote COVID-Ventilation Triage of Disabled Persons."

Chapter IV
Beneath the BMW's Wheels[1]

A large hand reaches out to me,
Up to me, beseeching me
In a gentrifying alleyway,
Strewn with needles and luxury vehicles.
The hand is thickened by scabrous lesions,
Inflammation, angry skin;
As blurred words slur "Sorry,"
"Not feeling well," "Help."
I reach for the hand and see a large man
Collapse further under parked wheels,
Before I could catch him,
Before I could ask him his name.

I kneel to better reach
The man beneath the wheels,
Take his hand, tell him "I've got you,"
"I'm going to help you," "I'm a doctor."
I place my left hand on his forehead,
Thickened with more torturous skin,
Sandwiching swollen eyes
Above roughened cheeks, remnants of beard,
And the tattered woollen collar
Of his not-warm-enough red plaid jacket,
Missing buttons on his chest,
Still wet from last night's weather.

I encourage him from beneath the wheels
For better air for him to breathe,
And for me to better assess
The texture of his infirmity.
His watery eyes greet mine,
I reassure, ask his name.
Lack-of-breath doesn't answer,
So I suggest if in pain
He nod his head, which he does,
As I explain he needs a hospital.
His troubles' tremble shakes my hand,
As the man nods again.

Just then a passerby
On his way to a Porsche,
Spits, "These guys clutter our lane,
And should be arrested of course."
And when behind his Porsche's
Clear-coated secure door,
Lowers a tinted window with,
"I'll call the police as I've done before,
But the police can't keep them
Off our streets;
Just tell me to ignore them,
But that's not easy. I park here."

I plead with the Porsche man,
"Please call an ambulance instead."
The man beneath the wheels
Squeezes my hand, nods his head.
But we don't trust the Porsche man,
Driving off, spraying slush;
So I let go of my touch, "Just for a minute,"
Find my phone, push 911.
When asked for the address
To which the ambulance should be sent,

I describe "An alley west of Parliament Street,
Just south of the apartments."

I'm put on hold for several minutes,
Then told, "Police were dispatched."
I demand, "This man needs an ambulance,
And I wouldn't have called if he didn't."
And add, "I'm a doctor,"
As I hear, "A car will be there."
So I cover the man with my winter coat,
And stroke his furrowed forehead.
The anguish of his blistered lips
Quiver, then whisper,
"Thanks," as he shivers,
As he waits, as he waits.

After too many too-long minutes,
A police car ambles the alley,
The policeman in it screaming,
"Get away from him! Are you crazy?
Do you have any idea
What that guy might have?"
I answer, "Yes, I'm a doctor,"
And hear, "Then you should know better."
He throws out the window,
"At least put on these gloves and mask."
I don't take them as the man's hand asks
To keep holding touch.

The policeman calls an ambulance
That bides its time before arriving;
Its mission for this person
Diverted by "indigent," less urgent.
The man is pulled from between the wheels,
Lifted on a stretcher, loaded in.
I ask permission to ride with him

To ensure he's looked after,
Rather than endure the long internment
Sentenced to invisible persons like him;
Persons seen as "indigent," "Indigenous," "chronic,"
Triaged from the focus of the too-few nurses.

But I'm denied permission to ride with him
And don't even ask where he'll be taken,
So I could meet the man there,
And ease his despair of waiting,
Curtained in some corner,
Ignored, enduring pain.
But I don't ask because I fear
The mire of the system,
And I'm a visitor here
With research to finish,
And know in this minute
I'm forever diminished by my silence.

I just stand frozen in the alley
Behind Parliament Street stores,
Watching an ambulance slush north
On its course to some Emerg;
An impotent physician
Letting down another patient,
With the excuse of, "Nothing I can do"
To limit my advocacy, my responsibility.
I greet others "like him"
Our systems have forgotten,
Bearing packed plastic bags,
Or pushing shopping carts with all they have.

I wonder what "they" must think
Of this path to paradise we inhabit,
Amidst sparkling new BMWs,
Porsches, and a Lexus;

And rich persons who park cars here,
Sharing the same pavement,
But wearing different vestments
That testament injustice
In a country that permits
A few having much too much,
And too many not near enough,
By any compassionate metric.

There are many such "neighbourhoods"
Where increasingly more
Persons are denied
By the widening divide
Of our unjust class system,
That we idealist students
Were sure we would eradicate,
But is now more firmly fabricated
By the tax breaks we once hated,
And the "trickle-down" philosophies,
Against which we demonstrated
While taking our degrees.

Physicians are prominent pistons
In the contagion of this erosion,
As seen in our frequent
Revolts against taxation.
Yet for those of us whose ethos
Cannot permit that on our watch,
"The system" we fought to fix,
With emphasis on social determinants,
Still exhibits lack of access,
Worsened by the two-tier erosion
Greater profits insist,
But social justice prohibits.

We must assist this new generation
Of social-conscious students
Be the conscience we've forgotten,
And the reignition of our once-vision,
To be "a just society,"[2]
First in health and social systems.
We must insist this realization
For the benefit of all Canadians,
So none will be left behind
Beneath a BMW's wheels,
For "None is too many"[3]
For any of us to conceal.

A modified version of the first section of this poem was published as the short story "Homeless Beneath a BMW's Wheels" in the Canadian Medical Association Journal *in 2020 (Nisker, 2020).*

---

1. *Beneath the Wheel*, the 1968 Hermann Hesse novel, explores his suppression under an archaic Swiss education system in the early 1900s. I borrow from Hesse's title to recount the injustice inflicted on socio-economically suppressed persons in Canada.
2. Pierre Trudeau, "Canada must be a just society," 1968.
3. A "senior Canadian official ... in early 1945, was asked how many Jews would be allowed into Canada after the war.... 'None,' he said, 'is too many'" (Troper & Abella, *None Is Too Many*, 1982, p. xix).

Chapter V
COVID Injustice Before I Heard the Word "COVID"

Even though I am a physician
I had not learned of the "virus of concern"
Even though the virus had been rampant
In Wuhan since the autumn[1]
Even though the virus gave me pneumonia
Before they gave the virus a name[2]
China had that successfully suppressed
Knowledge of the virus but not the virus

Opaque China became the secret epicentre[3]
Of a "super-spreader" event[4]
Rather than transparently alerting the world
To its contagious public health disaster
Camouflage banned viral social media
Prevented infected from entering hospitals
Instructed television to diminish importance[5]
Punished doctors who spoke of the virus[6]

Suppression of knowledge of the virus
Permitted unmasked distance-lacked air travel
To persist unabated around the globe
Transporting the virus along with people
Including the Sunwing flight to Mexico

For "Reading Week"[7] 2020
That incubated my partner and me
And likely the "virus of concern"

On our third morning in the sun
I succumbed to fever and coughing
And conceded to symptoms and partner's insistence
And was taken to the local physician
Who tapped my chest, whispered "deep breath"
As he listened to my lungs with concern
Softly told me "pneumonia"
And prescribed me antibiotics

Next morning my egregious coughing
Had so dramatically worsened
That my partner found a seat for me
On the next Sunwing back to Canada
In which there was no space to "social distance"
Before I learned the term "social distance"
So I pressed my head against a cold window
And asked the flight attendant for a mask

As it was rare to wear a mask then
The attendant could not find one
So the best I could do was dutifully cough
Into my wool sweater's sleeve
Between coughs I kept struggling
To inflate my fluid-filling lungs
With just limited success
I felt like I was drowning[8]

In the Customs Hall I plastered a wall
Till all passengers funnelled through
A security guard seeing my hesitancy
Asked me if there was a problem
I responded "I have pneumonia

And don't want to infect other passengers
Or you Sir for that matter"
He promptly backed away

I grabbed my bag from the dizzying carousel
Stepped into a cab, asked that windows be lowered
The driver resisted amidst frigid winter
But on hearing my first cough complied
Drowning waves swept over me
As the taxi neared my home
And I debated asking the driver
Continue three more blocks to the hospital

But my fear my colleagues there
Would insist me onto a ventilator
Caused my claustrophobia to reconsider
As it fears a ventilator more than death[9]
For I had made peace with death three years previous
Because of metastatic cancer[10]
So even in drowning's grip[11]
I let ventilator fear persist

Balance-trouble stumbled the walk
And fumbled my key into the front door's lock
And when it rotated I tumbled the door
To face plant the flagstone floor
I snaked the steps toward my bed
But on the fourth gasped for breath
Grasped my cell pressed 911
But not the call button yet

My partner called to check on me
I responded "fine" but breath betrayed
And though I insisted she remain
She boarded the next plane
And had just made it back

When she developed cough and fever
The following week we learned our virus
Would be termed COVID-19

1. Wuhan, China, had a massive outbreak in the fall of 2019 of the virus that
would be eventually named COVID-19 (World Health Organization, "WHO-
Convened Global Study of Origins of SARS-CoV-2," 2021).
2. The World Health Organization would name the virus COVID-19 (World
Health Organization, "WHO-Convened Global Study of Origins of SARS-CoV-
2," 2021).
3. China's neighbour, North Korea, would also become a secret epicenter, and
suppress knowledge of its COVID epidemic until May 2022 (Kim, "Nearly
10% of North Korea's Population Sick," 2022).
4. "Super spreader" is the term now used when gatherings beyond maximum
limits spread COVID contagion (Kolnes et al., "Estimating the Consequences
of a COVID-19 Super Spreader," 2022; Li et al., "Modeling the dynamics of
coronavirus with super-spreader class," 2022).
5. Filmmaker Nanfu Wang, *In the Same Breath*, 2021. Zeitchik, "A Scathing New
Documentary from HBO," 2021.
6. Zeitchik, "A Scathing New Documentary from HBO," 2021.
7. "Reading Week" is the misnomer for the vacation in February that universities
afford students (and professors), presumably to catch up on their work. A
Sunwing flight from Montreal to Mexico for "Reading Week" January 2022
amidst a COVID surge would achieve prominence in the Canadian press for the
twenty-somethings partying in the aisles, void of masks and social distancing
(Marchand, "Passengers on Sunwing Party Plane," 2022).
8. I have a morbid fear of drowning, as described in Chapter 3 of *Love and
Injustice in Medicine*, "I'm Sorry Ronnie" (Nisker, 2022). To obviate this fear, I
swim long distances in open water, which was the reason I was in Mexico for
our University's "Reading Week."
9. See Chapter III, "Claustrophobia's Fear of a COVID Ventilator."
10. See Chapter 25 of *Love and Injustice in Medicine*, "The Arrogance of 'But All
You Need Is a Good Index Finger'" (Nisker, 2022).
11. I reflect on my cousin's drowning in Chapter 3 of *Love and Injustice in
Medicine*, "I'm Sorry Ronnie" (Nisker, 2022).

Chapter VI
COVID Aggression Condemns a Muslim Family Near Our Medical School[1]

Post-chemo's fear of a COVID ventilator
Cloistered me from contagion in social distance shelters
Until tragedy found our University town
And unbound my COVID shackles to shoulder to shoulder kneel down
On blood-stained ground where a family had just been murdered
At the hate-sharpened end of a tire-skid scythe of black rubber
Where I throw blossoms from my garden on a flower volcano's eruption
And join hands with new friends who happen to be Muslim

Their families may have come from Lebanon or Pakistan
Or Saudi Arabia or Africa or Afghanistan or Kuwait
For a better fate for women free of misogynist hate
Did they now contemplate their migrate to Canada a mistake
And closer friends had come as "foreign medical graduates"[2]
To learn more medicine in order to become specialists
Did they now sense concern of appearing a bit foreign
Like they did after 911 because they happen to be Muslim

In our University town's multi-ethnic and educated fabric
It was easy to forget that beneath the surface white supremacists lurk
Even as we watched their horrific prejudice in Alberta and Quebec

And other provinces where some citizens for Muslims lack respect
Indeed are circumspect of all persons whose appearance is different
Whether the persons are Indigenous or Black or immigrant
Or living with disabilities or gay or lesbian or trans
Along with the persons who happen to be Muslim

The next day I entered the hospital where for many years I have practised
And where Intensive Care has expanded with the COVID-virus infected
As well as a nine-year-old boy with fractures and organ damage
From being plowed down by the hate-virus that infected a white supremacist
Who believed that killing Muslims would be so well received
He didn't need a balaclava nor white-hooded robe to attack a family
On their evening walk near our University where the boy's parents had studied
In a country they thought was free even if they happen to be Muslim

How do you tell a nine-year-old in an intensive care bed
When he asks where are his parents that his parents are dead
How do you submerge the murders of his sister and grandmother
Until he recovers enough to absorb the atrocity that occurred
How do you disguise from the eyes of a child full of goodness
That his family was murdered by hate purchased on the net
How can this child look forward to a future without the concern
That murder will capture him for the sin he happens to be Muslim

1. Western University is in London, Ontario, a few blocks from where this family was intentionally struck by a truck on June 6, 2021, and where the mother and father in this family achieved Master's degrees in physiotherapy. In the three months following the attack on this family, COVID-aggression was again exhibited in four sexual assaults (Dubinski, "Arrests Made after 4 Western Students Reported Sexual Assaults," 2021), and a manslaughter on Western's campus (Dolynny, "Second Person Wanted in Connection with Western Student's Death," 2021). I have also observed COVID-aggression when the cars and trucks of young men speed around the corner separating Western University from my home.
2. Pejoratively called "FMGs."

Chapter VII
Ruth

Calcedonies are rocks
Crusty-surfaced rocks
Rocks that open to onyx and amethyst
Chrysoprase and agate
To become amulets and talismans
Bookends and paper weights
For into each calcedony's core
Millennia poured melted magic

Calcedonies depend on humans
To endow them wisdom or courage
Healing powers or spiritual powers
Ferocity or peace
For each calcedony is unique
Speaks its singular dialect
Seeks its singular respect
As its dignity connects

Friends give Ruth calcedonies
Like the Spanish melon-size bookends
That have bookended her computer
Since her paper books ended
But her computer patiently waits[1]
For Ruth to press its power button

Just as it has waited each day for 17 years
After Ruth turned her last page

Ruth's bookends resemble
Her brain's magnetic resonance image
Complete with fluid-filled ventricles
And crenulated cerebral cortex
With white flecks that attest to the progress
Of the condition disconnecting
Ruth's brain from her voluntary muscles[2]
Except those that open her eyes and move her chin in all directions

Ruth's chin muscles permit her to speak
Albeit quietly and "rarely heard"[3]
And permit Ruth to eat
Albeit slowly and with assistance
And "more important" Ruth's chin muscles wave
The magic wand that propels her
The joystick on her powerchair
Her "chariot of disaster"

Ruth suffers pressure sores
Where her chair sandwiches her skin
Because she can't sense pressure "down there"
And shift her weight off the pressure
Pressure sores are often called bedsores
But Ruth takes umbrage with this word
And assures "My bed never gets sore"
When the word is uttered by doctors or nurses

When Ruth's pressure sores get infected
She is admitted for intravenous antibiotics
Ruth once asked a nurse to show her
What an infected bedsore looks like
The nurse needed two mirrors for Ruth to observe
Concentric circles of purple and black

And red and yellow "crud"
"Sort of an angry archery target"

When Ruth is with us and recovered enough
From the bedsore sepsis relentless in sending her here
Each day Ruth patiently waits[4]
To be lifted onto her powerchair
And have her chin Velcroed to its joystick
Then Ruth begins haunting the hospital halls
Hunting doctors at full throttle
Making a blood sport of it

When Ruth spots a doctor she halts her chair
Slowly moves her chin to turn its front wheels
In the direction of the doctor's white coat
As if it is a matador's red cape
She imagines her left foot[5] stamping bullring sand
Then Ruth pushes her chin forward
Charging at the matadoctor
A ferocious bull on wheels

Doctors never notice her charge
Because "patients are invisible to doctors"
But when Ruth is almost on one of us
Terror grips as we plaster the nearest wall
But unlike murderous matadors
Matadoctors never beckon a second charge
Though like matadors kill bulls in the end
Matadoctors killed Ruth in the end

Ruth's "life savings" bought a newer computer
That her chin could function through her chair's joystick
And "the latest in voice-activated software"
To write the poems collected in her heart
But Ruth needs a biomedical engineer
To connect her chin with her computer

And had been languishing on a three-year waiting list
When she drove her chair into my kneecaps

The next day I limp through the front door
Of our hospital's mammoth amphitheatre
Seconds before I am scheduled to begin
Our weekly "Monday Night Narratives" exploration[6]
However I am riveted by Ruth
Whose chair is proximate to the front door
The only door wheelchairs can enter
And then there are steps but no ramps

I feel pressure to begin but am confined by questions
How did Ruth talk a doctor into a "can leave ward" order
Or was no order ever written
And nurses are searching the hospital for her
How did Ruth learn of "Monday Night Narratives"
From a med student or nurse or a poster
How did Ruth know the amphitheatre's location
Was it from being displayed here over the years

I hear "Doc do you like my slippers"
And stare down at bear-paw slippers
I hear "Doc I've had these for years"
And fear Ruth is purposefully throwing me off
Of course slippers don't wear out when not walked on
Or was Ruth applauding the nurses for not losing them
I refocus and take a deep breath
"We have a guest with us tonight"

After the medical students leave
Ruth asks me to retrieve her cigarettes
From the sack on the back of her chair
I sigh "Let's go outside in the fresh air"
Nine feet[7] from the hospital I reluctantly agree
To place a cigarette in Ruth's lips

And carefully light it with four matches
Before Ruth takes a drag and asks me to write her story

Ruth tells me that a month previously
Sepsis spread through her body from an infected bedsore
And by the time an ambulance brought her to Emerg
She appeared unconscious to the doctors
But Ruth was not unconscious just too exhausted
To open her eyes or respond to questions
And as she couldn't feel them pinching her
She was unresponsive to painful stimuli[8]

Yet Ruth could hear them debate her fate
"Death with dignity or a persistent vegetative state"
A "bed-blocker" in our expensive care unit[9]
Intended for "higher quality of life"[10]
Ruth was concerned Quality of Life Assessments[11]
Could trap persons "like her" in lethal traps
So she considered an Advance Directive
That everything be done for her "no matter what"

But Ruth heard of danger with Advance Directives
And worried written words could be used against her
To foster her death with dignity
So she firmly reconsidered
Then Ruth heard of Life Story Decision-Making
For which you carry a card with contact information
Of persons you trust to make decisions for you
Ruth calls her card her "life preserver"

I come home from a distant conference
To see my phone's red light flashing
And hear my answering machine tremble
"Ruth's in trouble come to the hospital"
I assume the woman who called
Is on Ruth's list of trusted persons

Trusted to insist all be done for her
As Ruth wants "to live no matter what"

I drive urgently to the hospital
Leave my car at the ER doors
Dash in and look at "The Board"[12]
Ruth's name is not there
I ask to which floor she's been admitted
But their computer is taking too long
So I run up the stairs to Intensive Care
Worrying and hoping Ruth is there

The nurse at the desk seems to expect me
Her left index finger is pointing
To a draped-off bed at the Unit's far end
Where incandescent curtains project ominous shadows
I turn to run to the curtains
But the nurse grips my left wrist
And urges "Please stay with me
At least till they're finished"

I extricate my wrist and run
And fling open the curtains … to horror
Bacteria has necrosed Ruth's skin
And swollen her body to a huge balloon
Knotted at her neck and elbows and wrists
By a sadistic birthday-party clown
Ruth's closed eyes bulge black tennis balls
Ruth's chin is gone

The periphery of my underwater vision
Sees an ICU doc on my left
Acknowledging me as he draws
Lethal drugs into syringes
Hollowness expands within me
Vacuuming me downward

I fight the hollowness with *I can stop this*
Ruth wants "to live no matter what"

I focus hard at Ruth
Working hard to see
Working hard to breathe
Drowning in what I see
I notice a blurred woman sitting to my right
As I turn left to the ICU doctor
"You can't disconnect her
Ruth wants 'to live no matter what'"[13]

He puts his hand on my shoulder
Whispers "There's nothing left of her"
I retort "How can you be sure
Ruth has appeared dead before"
He turns my shoulders "Jeff look at her
There's nothing left of her"
I plead again "How can you be sure"
But he just goes back to his syringes

I put my body between Ruth's and his
As Ruth's Life Story Decision-Making suggests I should
But instead of insisting Ruth remain on the ventilator
I place my lips where Ruth's right ear should have been
I plead "Ruth give me a sign
Twitch an eyelid or move your chin
Try to move something
Help me Ruth please"

Earlier versions of Ruth's story were published as the short story "Chalcedonies" in the Canadian Medical Association Journal,[14] *and in* From the Other Side of the Fence: Stories from Health Care Professionals.[15] *I then expanded Ruth's story to a full-length play that was produced in several countries, and published in my compilation* From Calcedonies to Orchids[16]

as well as chapters in Reflective Practice,[17] *and* Health Humanities Reader.[18]
I was able to honour Ruth better with the novel Patiently Waiting For....[19]

---

1. *Patiently Waiting For...* is the title of the novel Ruth encouraged me to write about her (Nisker, 2015).
3. Voluntary muscles are the muscles we can control.
4. The exact words of the woman I call Ruth appear in quotation marks.
5. *Patiently Waiting For...* is the title of the novel Ruth encouraged me to write about her (Nisker, 2015).
6. I specifically have Ruth imagine she uses "her left foot" in homage to the play *My Left Foot* by Christy Brown, which was made into the Oscar-winning film of the same name directed by Jim Sheridan and starring Daniel Day-Lewis.
7. "Monday Night Narratives" was a two hour interactive program I started in 1996 to "imbue compassion in medical students" (Nisker, 1997).
8. Nine feet is the distance to where a person can smoke as posted on a sign. Ruth stopped her powerchair right in front of the sign.
9. Pinching and needling skin are part of a standard neurological assessment to determine "response to painful stimuli."
10. The "Expensive Care Unit" is the term too often used by physicians in a semi-derogatory manner for the Intensive Care Unit.
11. "Higher quality of life" became the triage consideration for ICU admission during the COVID-19 pandemic. See Chapter II, "Webinar Physicians' Cavalier Terms Promote COVID-Ventilation Triage of Disabled Persons."
12. "Quality of Life Assessments," lightly called "qualies" by some Emerg and ICU physicians, residents, and even medical students, predict the worth of living a disabled condition through the eyes of "able-bodied" assessors on tick box and short answer paper.
13. "The Board" occupied a wall with the names of persons "patiently waiting" in the ER during various stages, including: "waiting" to be seen by a physician, "waiting" to have blood drawn, "waiting" to receive results of their blood tests, "waiting" to be sent to radiology, "waiting" to receive X-ray results, "waiting" to be referred to a specialist, "waiting" to be admitted, and "waiting" to be sent home (Nisker, *Patiently Waiting*, 2015).
14. See Chapter 20 of *Love and Injustice in Medicine*, "Webinar Physicians' Cavalier Terms for COVID-Ventilator Triage of Disabled Persons" (Nisker, 2022).
15. Nisker, "Chalcedonies," *Canadian Medical Association Journal*, 2001.
16. Nisker, "Chalcedonies," *From the Other Side of the Fence*, 2008.
17. Nisker, *From Calcedonies to* Orchids, 2012.
18. Nisker, "Calcedonies," *Reflective Practice*, 2010.
19. Nisker, "Calcedonies," *Health Humanities Reader*, 2014.
20. Nisker, *Patiently Waiting For...* 2015.

Chapter VIII
Antivaxxer Xenophobic
COVID Violence

Antivaxxers' COVID violence from defiance of vaccine
Condemns innocent persons to ventilator prisons
And even suffocation and other horrid death sentences
Because of the contagion[1] of antivaccination propaganda

Antivaxxers also spread contagion of opposition to Public Health regulation
And other mandates put in place to keep vulnerable persons safe[2]
And curb the surge of COVID's next scourge
And the "fallout"[3] of its radiation through our post-restriction nation[4]

Antivaxxers are clogging our intensive care units
"Occupying"[5] 70 percent[6] of "expensive care"[7] beds
Bed blockers[8] of persons with no alternative but be there
But COVID's flood prevents their enter through this life-preserver door

Antivaxxers' venomous rhetoric super-spreads[9] misinformation
On the side effects of vaccination and its mandate's motivation
Selfishness sublimating any sniff of community consciousness
Violent verbiage "trumping"[10] any logic of vaccination

Antivaxxers applaud themselves as courageous risk-takers
But the lives they courageously risk are usually the lives of others
Including nurses and doctors pushed past our previous limits
Because hours of work are not infinite nor steps to protect us from COVID

Antivaxxer truckers are clogging our streets[11]
Blatantly blaring air horns of right-wing beliefs
Seen in brazen waving of swastika rags
And Confederate flags of slavery's past and KKK hate to this day[12]

Antivaxxer truckers[13] take hostages on highways and border crossings[14]
In the name of the glorious purpose of personal "freedom"[15]
But what antivaxxers really mean when they loudly espouse "freedom"
Is "freedom" of persons with similar belief systems

Antivaxxer arrogance leads many Canadians to believe
That opposition to vaccination is an acceptable alternative
To community consciousness and moral responsibility
To protect others from disease no matter what doctrine we believe[16]

---

1. An increase in COVID deaths and morbidities was reported for persons with disabilities in Canada (Brown et al., "Outcomes in Patients with and without Disability," 2022).
2. In the prescient film *Contagion* (2011), directed by Steven Soderbergh, Kate Winslet portrays a public health physician who uncovers a lethal virus spreading in the Chicago region. This physician dies from the virus after taking swabs from numerous patients.
3. I grew up during the Cold War under the threat of radiation fallout from Russian nuclear attack.
4. In April 2022, subsequent to the loosening of restrictions, a "sixth" wave of COVID began killing Canadians (CBC News, April 2022).
5. "Occupy" was proclaimed by the antivaxxer truckers and others who took over the streets in Ottawa, Canada's capital, from January 28 to February 20, 2022, in a manner similar to when President Trump encouraged Americans to "occupy" the capital building of the Congress of the United States on January 6, 2021 (Reston & Liptak, "The Day America Realized How Dangerous Donald Trump Is," 2021). There had previously been an "occupy" movement in Toronto and other Canadian cities in 2011, protesting the global financial system, as well as economic and social inequality (Habib, "Occupy Canada Rallies Spread in Economic 'Awakening'," 2011).
6. More than 70 percent of persons in Canada's ICUs were unvaccinated in January 2022 (Daigle, "In this Ontario Hospital, It's Mostly the Unvaccinated Who Are Overwhelming the ICU," 2022; Favaro & Jones, "Inside an ICU Where 70 Per Cent of COVID-19 Patients Are Unvaccinated," 2022).

7. The term "expensive care" is commonly used by physicians when referring to the intensive care unit.

8. "Bed blocker" (Styrborn & Thorslund, "Delayed Discharge of Elderly Hospital Patients," 1993; McGrail et al., "The Quick and the Dead," 2001; Green, Croskerry & Rieck, "Bed Blocker," 2020) is the pejorative term too often used by physicians for persons whose likelihood of coming out of the ICU with "quality of life" may be limited. See Chapter II, "Webinar Physicians' Cavalier Terms Promote COVID-Ventilation Triage of Disabled Persons"; also see Chapter VII, "Ruth."

9. "Super spreader" is the term used for gatherings beyond the maximum limits that risk COVID-contagion from person to person (Kolnes et al., "Estimating the Consequences of a COVID-19 Super Spreader," 2022; Li et al., "Modeling the Dynamics of Coronavirus with Super-Spreader Class," 2022).

10. I use the term "trumping" because on February 24, 2022, former–U.S. president Trump condemned Canada's COVID restrictions (CBC News). In addition, Trump supporters cheered the Canadian trucker convoys opposing our vaccine mandate (Tasker, "Thousands Opposed to COVID-19 Rules Converge on Parliament Hill," 2022; "COVID-19 Protesters Demonstrate across Canada in Support of Truck Convoy in Ottawa," 2022). "Trumping" is a term used in card games like bridge when cards of one of the four "suits" (e.g., diamonds) become endowed with the power to be superior to other "suits."

11. "COVID-19 Protesters Demonstrate across Canada in Support of Truck Convoy in Ottawa," 2022; Tasker, "Thousands Opposed to COVID-19 Rules Converge on Parliament Hill," 2022.

12. The "Stars and Bars" was the Confederate flag during the American Civil War, in which Southern pro-slavery advocates proclaimed the "freedom" of "The Confederacy" after President Lincoln's anti-slavery Emancipation Declaration on January 1, 1863. This flag proudly flew over the State Legislature Building in South Carolina until it was finally lowered in 2021.

13. In no way is this poem intended to sully the reputation of truckers, as my Grandfather, with whom we lived when I was young, was a trucker, and my admiration and respect for him grew after I read the trucker scene in John Steinbeck's *The Grapes of Wrath* (1939).

14. Lord, "Trucker Convoy," 2022. Antivaxxer truckers occupied Canada's capital, Ottawa, for three weeks ("The Convoy Crisis in Ottawa: A Timeline of Key Events," 2022), and blocked border crossings to the United States at Windsor, Ontario (Fraser, "Ambassador Bridge Reopens," 2022); Emerson, Manitoba ("Protesters Continue to Blockade Major Canada-U.S. Border Crossing in Manitoba", 2022); and Coutts, Alberta ("Frustration Mounts as Blockade Snarling Access to U.S. Border Continues at Alberta Port of Entry", 2022).

15. Tasker, "Thousands Opposed to COVID-19 Rules Converge on Parliament Hill," 2022.

16. James Dwyer of Canada's Memorial University brings to our attention on February 3, 2022, the writings of John Stuart Mill, who Dwyer considers "the greatest champion of individual liberty" and "individuals' right to regulate their

own lives when their actions do not impinge on others." Dwyer argues that Mill "comes to the view that people's conduct should only be restricted when it violates a distinct duty to another person or to the public." Dwyer suggests that protecting others "is what ultimately justifies vaccine requirements, limitations on public gatherings, mask mandates, and other measures."

Chapter IX
She Lived with the Knowledge

She lived with the knowledge it would happen to her
Knowledge more felt than understood
Knowledge gleaned from intuition that could not be confessed
Knowledge that always lived and never rests.
She lived with the knowledge it would happen to her
Woke each day to the knowledge it would happen to her
That what happened to her Mother would happen to her
She only wondered when it would happen and when would it end.

My knowledge began with my Grandmother
With whom I lived at my life's beginning
Who lived with us at her life's ending
My wonderful second mother.
Powdered in kitchen-table flour
She told stories of Schweitzer and Hammarskjöld
Patiently engraving her goodness
To proxy me with their purpose.

Breast cancer found my Grandmother when she was fifty-four
I was sixteen when she died a few years later
I did not know my Grandmother had breast cancer
I did not know she would soon die.
Though she suffered surgery and chemotherapy
Radiation and fluid taps

They were carefully hidden behind parental backs
Forbidden to my adolescent distraction.

But perhaps those backs were less opaque
And it was I who willingly chose to take
Each molecule of selfish density to deny
Truth to a teenager too enamoured with teenage rise.
Even when my Grandmother moved in with us
And lived in a hospital bed in my room
I forbid contemplation of where that bed led
Till my Grandmother was led to a hospice hospital.

A few days later my Mother's telephone whisper
"Jeff, come to the hospital but don't tell your Brother or Sister"
Insisted it would be the last time
My Grandmother's eyes and mine would entwine.
Yet as I held her goodness in my hand
It was the first time our eyes entwined in her truth
We stared hard at each other
Long after the "Visitors' Hours are over."

I could not contemplate leaving her
Because she would never leave me
As long as I held the hand that held me
The hand that still holds me.
I wore her colours in this joust with injustice
And would not be unseated
Till "too young" rules decreed I must get up
And my trust of justice was lanced forever.

I loved my Grandmother very much
For years I daily grieved
But never for one moment perceived
That what happened to my Grandmother would happen to her.
Seven years later medical print premonished
My Mother would suffer the same injustice

The fact soon fell from its suspended shelf
When my Mother discovered her assassin herself.

It had been only two months since
The mammogram I arranged proclaimed "all clear"
My Mother bravely bore her long-accepted bier
And missioned to soften her family's fear.
Mastectomy delivered a tiny stone
The surgeon delivered an optimistic poem
"No spread, no further treatment to tread"
But the pathology report delivered an "aggressive" retort.

This surgeon shared "aggressive" with just the physician-son
As it was a time when cancer-patient families
Were encouraged to cheery possibilities
Through tones that knell "All's well."
The physician to physician share
Of all may not be well
Was a care I reluctantly did not share
With my pleasantly pastelled family.

The tumour's small size and negative nodes
Bode no tamoxifen, no radiation, no chemo
Tamoxifen was new then and thought to later lend
Leukemia to women it borrowed from breast cancer.
Radiation and chemo would hurl her further abuse
I could not advocate their adjuvant use
Not when the sure surgeon's words of optimism
So soothed my reassured family.

I abrogated "aggressive" awareness
And acquiesced my Mother to another's care
I let the surgeon take command, and went to California
On a breast cancer research fellowship.
Of course I now admonish this acquiescence
I should have spent her each remaining day

Finding ways to repay the love she lavished
But my Mother would not hear of it.

A year later my Father's long-distance words
"Jeff I have some bad news"
Collapsed my knees, my lungs, my life
As it confessed the poison she possessed.
Nothing further needed to be said
I knew my Mother would soon be dead
My silence heard my Father urge chemo would cure her
A reassurance irrelevant to my Mother's reality.

I flew home viewing 8 mm movies of my Mother
There were so many smiles in so few years
No sound was needed to feel her embrace
No colour required to feel her grace.
My friends likened my Mother to Maria in *West Side Story*
But I view my Mother as more beautiful
Eyes smiling on a dance floor as she spins beneath my arm
Eyes in love as she wraps herself in my Father's arms.

I hurried the hospital's revolving door
Then sped the elevator to the cancer floor
Where its doors opened on a black "In Loving Memory"
Engraving the names of the cancer-killed.
I quickly glanced at my Grandmother's golden name
Avoiding noticing the black space below
That would soon be embossed with the engraving
Of my Mother's so-golden name.

I ran fast to the nurses' station
Breathlessly begging my Mother's room number
I ran faster to that room and parted the curtains
Only to find a woman who was not my Mother.
The woman smiled at me warmly
Her head bare in a wheelchair

I said "Sorry" and bolted to the room next door
Before being locked in the abhor that I had just spoken to my Mother.

Panic punished as I tried to undo my betrayal
I ran back to her room to her unvanquished smile
To her "Don't worry you didn't recognize me without my hair"
I hugged her waist with my head and begged her forgiveness.
My Mother locked her fingers in the curls of my hair
And quickly released me to her comfort
My sobs flooded my Mother's gown
Where I felt I had drowned.

With each week's advance my family firmed their faith
That more chemo would turn metastatic cancer's advance
Sympathetic nurses encouraged this not-credible credulity
I of course knew no such even temporary luxury.
I silently shouldered death's imminent answer
As cancer poured its spores through my Mother
Growing tubes to remove its seditious sap
From her abdomen, her bladder, her brain, her back.

Soon the cancer that seeded her brain
Convulsed her diminishing body
The doctors countered with their sweet sedation
That took her from us before we were ready.
I asked the drugs be backed off to bring my Mother back
And her crystal comburence warmed another month
Till rare became the moments my Mother was aware
Of the love that surrounded her, the love she put there.

My family denied my Mother's imminent death
Constantly advising of the latest newspaper finds
Such as Laetrile and other unevidenced medicines
That were popular in the press at that time.
My gentle urge that there was no magic cure
In the world that could miracle my Mother

Was met with contempt and haranguing
That my heart had been hardened in medical training.

The elevator doors opened for the last time
The "In Loving Memory" list embossed my imminent loss
My eyes tunnelled to resist my Grandmother's golden name
And the space where my Mother's name would soon embrace hers.
My Grandfather met me near the elevator to eagerly effuse
"There's a new drug on the news that is sure to cure your Mother"
I hugged his helplessness and walked him to my Uncle and Aunt
Pacing the verandah to the vigil I would enter for the last time.

As my Mother began her terminal-breathing pattern
My Sister wept on my Mother's chest
My Father sat in a chair staring at his forever love
Glad her suffering would soon be over.
My Brother and I stood bookending her bed
Staring down at the kerchiefed head we so loved
Silent centurions guarding the gates of the dead
Steadfast in prohibiting our Mother's passage.

As I took my Mother's wedding-ringed left hand
My Brother took her right hand
We were touching an angel's gossamer wings
As they slowly spread for flight.
When her final breath exhaled her death
My Brother commenced cardiac massage
I refrained his wrists in whispered gauze
"She's gone but she will never leave us."

His eyes glazed over but mine could not
I lifted them to my Father's searching mine for what he already knew
We stared at each other for more than a long time
Longing for her, allies in loss.
My eyes turned back to Mother's eyes
Closed in peaceful sleep for eternity

I held my Mother's hand past cold[1]
I still hold her hand and will forever.

I love my Grandmother very much
I love my Mother very much
I love my Sister very much
Who lives with the knowledge it will happen to her,
Her knowledge is more felt than understood
Her knowledge gleaned from intuition that cannot be confessed
Her knowledge that always lived
Her knowledge that it will never rest.

She lives with the knowledge it will happen to her
Wakes each day to the knowledge it will happen to her
That what happened to her Grandmother will happen to her
That what happened to her Mother will happen to her.
She wonders when it will happen
She wonders when it will end
But "it" will not happen to my Sister
"It" will not happen to her daughters.

To prevent "it" from happening to sisters and daughters in other families, I wrote the play Sarah's Daughters *for public education regarding BRCA gene mutation breast cancer in the late 1990s. "She Lived with the Knowledge" had just been written in response to the request of Cancer Care Ontario to write a poem to be read at the opening ceremonies of its Annual Conference.* Sarah's Daughters *is a 90-minute play incorporating scientific information about BRCA gene mutations, and about the prevention, diagnosis and treatment of BRCA-related breast and ovarian cancer, including offering knowledge of the existence of this gene to women at risk.*[1]

Sarah's Daughters *drew on events that occurred in Canada regarding the lack of availability of testing for this gene, which remained confined to a research protocol long after it was clinically available in other countries. Further, the research protocol ignored the fact that the highest risk group, Jewish women whose ancestry was from Eastern Europe, was less likely to have an adequate number of women with breast cancer in their families to qualify them for testing. By focusing on the story of one woman, her family and her best friend, the play also aimed to place the ethical, health policy, and scientific issues in a context that was accessible and engaging for the general public. The play* Sarah's Daughters *(into which I morphed "She Lived with the Knowledge" as act I, scene 1) draws attention to the unjust gatekeeping policy that restricted most women at high risk of developing hereditary breast/ovarian cancer from accessing genetic counselling in Canada.*

Sarah's Daughters *toured Canada multiple times, as well as touring four other countries. It was performed for thousands of women, many of whom likely had a high hereditary risk of early onset breast cancer and were attracted by the theatre posters and other advertisement indicating the subject matter of the play.*

---

1. Nisker, *From Calcedonies to Orchids*, 2012.

Chapter X
Victor

Victor was a gentle giant
The strongest and kindest man
My hand ever met
My heart will never forget
Victor's strength was genetic
Augmented by farm childhood and welder adulthood
Victor's kindness was nongenetic
Yet the dominant ingredient of his nature

Victor's immense strength
Combined with his comburent kindness
To anoint him the point person
For his many family members and friends
Whenever they needed assistance
Be it in building a shed in their yard
Or brightening their spirits with hospital visits
Victor's presence was consistent

Victor's chronic welding tank
Collapsed discs in his lower back
Condemning walking to excruciating
And lifting to more than mortal
But Victor's strength carried the pain
Always remaining there for others

Yet I never appreciated Victor's strength
Until he carried pancreatic cancer

When two of Victor's older siblings
Suffered pancreatic cancer
There was suppressed suspicion
This cancer ran in Victor's family
But when his younger sister was diagnosed
It became too clear to Roxanne and me
That Victor's family carried a dominant gene
That doomed half of each generation

Victor never complained
Of the growing pain lancinating his core
Even when family members observed
Victor's skin had turned yellow
And strongly encouraged Victor
To see his family doctor
Who ordered a CAT scan that concurred
Victor's burden of pancreatic cancer

Victor was referred to a surgeon
Who assured the tumour's location
Blocking the bile duct causing jaundice
Declared cancer early enough for "cure"
A word too rarely heard
For quiet pancreatic cancer
But with this potential for "cure"
Victor endured a "Whipple's" procedure

"Whipple's" is perhaps the most onerous
Of all cancer surgeries
And Victor's took more hours
Than the surgeon had planned for
And on leaving the OR
He reported to Victor's family

That the cancer was more "aggressive"
Than anticipated prior to surgery

The surgeon's word "aggressive"
Reported to me urgently long-distance
Echoed another surgeon's word "aggressive"
Reported to me calmly in person
Outside the OR where my Mother endured
The mastectomy assured to "cure" her[1]
Victor's surgeon's word "aggressive"
Reverberated a similar death knell

Victor's strength insisted rapid recovery
To soon resume his daily rounds
Of assisting friends and family members
Till Victor's cancer soon recurred
And Victor's strength had to endure
The wrath of metastatic cancer's advance
Through his abdomen and liver
Strength I knew I would never have[2]

Victor generously gave me the gift
Of his person even when bothering him
On a calm Algonquin dock
While he was serenely trying to fish
This is my infinite portrait of Victor
On the quiet end of that dock
Fishing rod over the water
Patiently breathing the blissful peace

This visage of Victor permeates me
With radiance every day
His smile never diminishing with my questions
Always broadening when he brought in a bass
And Victor's smile broadened further
When I asked about hockey's "Uke Line"

Consisting of his Ukrainian heroes
Victor is my all-ethnic hero

I have a photograph of Victor
Holding two large fish on a dock
It sits beside my Mother's picture
And a quadriptych of Roxanne
Taken in Jasper by her sister
The Thanksgiving Victor knew was his last
And decided to give thanks
To the wife and daughters he loved

In the four pictures vertical mounted
Roxanne's face is in close profile
Almost kissing the grey-whiskered dandelion
She so delicately holds
In the first picture Roxanne is inhaling
In the second her cheeks grow to blow
In the third the dandelion's stem
Bends in the breeze of her breath

In the fourth picture her lips purse
In a mixture of smile and concern
Before she kisses the last whiskers
And sends these seeds to earth
Roxanne is making another wish
Another love-filled wish for Victor
A wish for delaying her Father's departure
A wish for retaining her Father's love

I had the gift of making it to Victor's hospital bed
The evening before he died
And taking his intravenoused right hand
Carefully and tenderly in mine
Then I received another gift from Victor
As he slowly opened his eyes

And embraced me in the warmth of his smile
Finding the strength amidst pain and sedation

In the years since Victor left us
I have been haunted by the fear
That I will not handle cancer's ravage
Nearly as well as Victor
And once shared this fear with Roxanne
Whose silence confirmed my fear's validity
"I'm not as strong as your Dad
I wish I was but I know I'm not"

As I am writing this poem of Victor
His niece is succumbing to pancreatic cancer
She is the exact age of Roxanne
And I am concerned for Roxanne
And upset with the reluctance
To fund research on hereditary pancreatic cancer
Because it is a rare form of cancer
Though the second most common cancer-killer

Victor will remain forever
The strongest man I ever met
Yet it was his gentleness that created
The tiny twig sculpture that graces my home
Reminiscing a tree bare of leaves
Standing up to a strong wind
A tree reminiscing Victor
A tree in which I believe

I know I never will possess
Victor's enduring strength
And know I will try but fail
To possess Victor's enormous kindness
And I am thankful for being granted
Extra years with Victor's miniature

Extra years with his giant presence
Extra years with the gift of Victor

---

1. See Chapter 10, "She Lived with the Knowledge" (Nisker, *Love and Injustice in Medicine*, 2022).
2. See Chapter 25, "The Arrogance of 'But All You Need is a Good Index Finger'" (Nisker, *Love and Injustice in Medicine*, 2022).

Chapter XI
Just Because "ICUs Have the Capacity"[1]

Our business-assisted Premier
Contrary to Public Health's wishes[2]
Declared "We're open for business"[3]
Because "ICUs have the capacity"[4]
To handle the anticipated increase
In COVID admissions they will see
And he was giving permission
For our economy to keep growing

Just because "ICUs have the capacity"
To absorb more COVID-inflicted persons
Is not a reason to sentence more therein
For the consideration of business
Not to mention for the purpose
Of assuring an election win
With a magnificent majority of citizens
Supporting his freedom decisions

But not supporting our vulnerable citizens
Because an ICU is no location to live in
Or die in as often happens
But should not happen with COVID
Let alone happen for the greater glory

Of an "open for business" Premier
And a Province free of the nuisance
Of COVID restrictions' inhibition of freedom

We must persist with precautions
Rather than be optimistic in believing
"ICUs have the capacity"
And always will have COVID capacity
To keep alive those who would not be there
If our Premier cared more for
His socio-disadvantaged constituents
Than the better-off citizens who elected him

---

1. Premier Doug Ford, April 2021, CBC News.
2. *Ibid*, CBC News.
3. *Ibid*, CBC News.
4. *Ibid*, CBC News.

Chapter XII
Our Third COVID Summer

In our third COVID summer
"COVID fatigue" sets in
So politicians lift restrictions
Before Public Health gives permission
As it appears in politicians' best interests
To soothsayer[1] COVID is "in the rear-view mirror"
A falsehood to foster "Open for Business"[2]
And summer pleasure for future voters

In our third COVID summer
The calm before autumn's COVID prediction
Has become fodder for ignoring
Public Health's dire warning
As we bask in "catch-up" celebrations
That lack masks and social distance
Applauded by our relaxed Premier
Because our ICUs can handle more COVID

In our third COVID summer
Our Premier applauds
Our "high vaccination rate"
As an excuse to remove the mask mandate
But COVID vaccines are not potent
And ICUs no place to live in

Or die in as many will in the autumn
With or without vaccination

In our third COVID summer
Variants breed beneath the surface
Not causing symptoms severe enough
For hospital admissions
Thus evidence for statisticians
To convince Business-elected politicians
To insist on masks and social distance
To diminish autumn's COVID

In our third COVID summer
I fear my grandchildren now consider me
The masked Poppa Jeff
Standoffish for some reason
As I no longer lift them in the air
To kiss their squealing belly buttons
Nor let them trampoline my abdomen
To spring their gorgeous giggles

In our third COVID summer
Rather I see confusion in my grandchildren's eyes
When they see my eyes above a mask
Instead of seeing the me who loves them dearly
But whose immunity is diminished
By chemotherapy's gift
Of extra years with grandchildren's laughter
Though COVID diminishes another summer

In our third COVID summer
The removal of mask mandates
From most spaces in our nation
Causes COVID complacency
But also COVID paranoia for the older
Including me when I face breathing on my masked face

Or the mask straps on my neck
At maskless clusters of check-out counters

In our third COVID summer
My triple-vaxxed Brother called
To let me know he has COVID
And was wasting his summer with cough
And on CBC television I learned
Our triple-vaxxed Prime Minister has COVID
As does the triple-vaxxed Prime Minister of the United Kingdom
And the triple-vaxxed President of the United States

In our third COVID summer
A proliferation of COVID aggression[3]
Spawns placards in bank windows
ABUSE OF TELLERS WILL NOT BE TOLERATED
But there are no signs on roads that warn
DANGER COVID-AGGRESSIVE DRIVERS
Who cut in and out of traffic
And are more dangerous than the COVID virus

In our third COVID summer
I also observe COVID aggression when I run
Close to the curb as per usual
But now hear profanity hurled
Through car windows speeding by
Or amplified at stop signs
Both with the addition of a certain finger
Though we're in COVID together

In our third COVID summer
"Dare I eat a peach"[4] of patio dining
With servers no longer masking
My answer is "Yes please"
For we need to go on living
While hoping "opening" won't increase dying

Before winter moves servers indoors
And clusters more maskless COVID

In our third COVID summer
"Big Pharma" promises new vaccines
Guaranteed to finally work
But we've heard this optimism before
And Omicron's variants will likely morph faster
Than scientists can pursue them
And will definitely spread faster
When there are no masks for inhibition

As colder weather suggests autumn
I let my guard down like many others
Before winter insists further reclusiveness
Which will again force me from our hospital
And its intimacy of "in-person"
Meetings and teachings and learnings
Onto Zoom, which is less human
By Chi-square significance

---

1. A "soothsayer" in Ancient Greek Mythology predicted the future often based on the throwing of small bones like dice, or observing how steam plumed from throwing water on hot stones.
2. The word "Business" was used frequently by Business-elected Ontario Premier Doug Ford in slogans like "We're open for Business." I capitalize "Business" because Ford presents it as a deity we need to worship.
3. COVID was claimed as the reason for more aggressive behaviours of males including a dramatic increase in the incidence of rape (CBC National News, August 2, 2022).
4. T.S. Elliot, *The Love Song of J. Alfred Prufrock*, 1915.

References

Introduction

"Mass Shooting in Buffalo, N.Y., That Killed 10 a Racially Motivated Hate Crime, Authorities Say." CBC News (May 14, 2022). https://www.cbc.ca/news/world/buffalo-grocery-store-shooting-1.6453755.

"What We Know about the Uvalde, Texas, Shooting Victims." CBC News (May 25, 2022). https://www.cbc.ca/news/world/uvalde-shooting-victims-1.6464874.

Fraser, K. "Ambassador Bridge Reopens with Heavy Police Presence Around Former Windsor, Ont., Protest Site." CBC News, February 14, 2022. https://www.cbc.ca/news/canada/windsor/ambassador-bridge-reopens-monday-1.6350729.

Nisker, J. "Philip." *Canadian Medical Association Journal* 168(6) (2003): 746–47.

Nisker, J. "She Lived with the Knowledge." *Ars Medica* 1(1) (2004): 75–80.

Nisker, J. "Chalcedonies." In *From the Other Side of the Fence: Stories from Health Care Professionals*, edited by J. Nisker, 172–76. Halifax: Pottersfield Press, 2008.

Nisker, J. "Calcedonies: Critical Reflections on Writing Plays to Engage Citizens in Health and Social Policy Development." *Reflective Practice* 11(4) (2010): 417–32.

Nisker, J. *From Calcedonies to Orchids: Plays Promoting Humanity in Health Policy*. Toronto: Iguana Books, 2012.

Nisker, J. "Calcedonies." In *Health Humanities Reader,* edited by T. Jones, D. Wear, and L.D. Friedman, Chapter 42. New Brunswick, NJ: Rutgers University Press, 2014.

Nisker, J. *Patiently Waiting For...* Toronto: Iguana Books, 2015.

Nisker, J.A. "Chalcedonies." *Canadian Medical Association Journal* 164(1) (2001): 74–75.

Nisker, J.A. "Narrative Ethics in Health Care." In *Toward a Moral Horizon,* edited by R. Starzomski, 285–309. Toronto: Pearson Education Canada Inc., 2004.

Nisker, J.A. "Orchids: Not Necessarily a Gospel." In *Mappa Mundi: Mapping Culture/Mapping the World,* edited by J. Murray, 61–110. Windsor: University of Windsor Press, 2001.

Nisker, J., and V. Bergum. "A Child on Her Mind." In *Mother Life Studies of Mothering Experience,* edited by V. Bergum and J. Van Der Zalm, 364–98. Edmonton: Pedagon Publishing, 2007.

Siegelman, J.N. "Reflections of a COVID-19 Long Hauler." *JAMA* 324(20) (November 24, 2020):2031–32. doi: 10.1001/jama.2020.22130. PMID: 33175108.

World Health Organization. "WHO-Convened Global Study of Origins of SARS-CoV-2: China Part [Internet]." World Health Organization (January 14–February 10, 2021). https://www.who.int/publications/i/item/who-convened-global-study-of-origins-of-sars-cov-2-china-part.

Chapter I—Confined to the COVID Sidelines

Brown, D. "Unions Fire Back at LHSC Boss's 'Shaming' over COVID-19 Protocol Lapses." *London Free Press* (2020). https://lfpress.com/news/local-news/unions-fire-back-at-lhsc-bosss-shaming-over-covid-19-protocol-lapses.

Dolynny, T. "Second Person Wanted in Connection with Western Student's Death." CBC News, September 17, 2021. https://www.cbc.ca/news/canada/london/second-person-wanted-in-connection-with-western-student-s-death-1.6180684.

Dubinski, K. "Arrests Made after 4 Western Students Reported Sexual Assaults in Past Week, University Official Says." CBC News, September 13, 2021. https://www.cbc.ca/news/canada/london/western-campus-sexual-violence-reports-1.6173443.

Newcombe, D. "Sudden Departure of Two LHSC Executives Might Cost $750,000 in Severance." CTV News (2021). https://london.ctvnews.ca/sudden-departure-of-two-lhsc-executives-might-cost-750-000-in-severence-1.5464633.

Shakespeare, William. *Richard III*. 1594.

Chapter II—Webinar Physicians' Cavalier Terms Promote COVID-Ventilation Triage of Disabled Persons

Dawidowicz, L. *The War Against the Jews 1933–1945*. New York: Holt, Rinehart & Winston, 1975.

Chapter III—Claustrophobia's Fear of a COVID Ventilator

Ballingall, A. "Former Huronia Residents Join Speakers' Series to Educate Others on Horrors Endured." *Toronto Star*, February 10, 2016. https://www.thestar.com/news/gta/2016/02/10/former-huronia-residents-join-speakers-series-to-educate-others-on-horrors-endured.html.

Battersby, S.J. "Huronia Survivors Work through Their Pain in Theatre Production." *Toronto Star*, April 13, 2018. https://www.thestar.com/news/gta/2016/05/31/huronia-survivors-work-through-their-pain-in-theatre-production.html

John Hopkins University of Medicine. "COVID-19 Dashboard." John Hopkins University of Medicine. Accessed March 28, 2022. https://coronavirus.jhu.edu/map.html

Marlin, Beth. "A Chance for Huronia's 'Invisible' to Be Seen and Heard." *Globe and Mail*, 2010.

Nisker, J. "Calcedonies: Critical Reflections on Writing Plays to Engage Citizens in Health and Social Policy Development." *Reflective Practice* 11(4) (2010): 417–32.

Nisker, J. "Calcedonies." In *Health Humanities Reader,* edited by T. Jones, D. Wear, and L.D. Friedman, Chapter 42. New Brunswick, NJ: Rutgers University Press, 2014.

Nisker, J. "Chalcedonies." In *From the Other Side of the Fence: Stories from Health Care Professionals,* edited by J. Nisker, 172–76. Halifax: Pottersfield Press, 2008.

Nisker, J. *From Calcedonies to Orchids: Plays Promoting Humanity in Health Policy.* Toronto: Iguana Books, 2012.

Nisker, J. *Patiently Waiting For...* Toronto: Iguana Books, 2015.

Nisker, J.A. "The Yellow Brick Road of Medical Education." *Canadian Medical Association Journal* 156(5) (1997): 689–91. https://www.ncbi.nlm.nih.gov/pubmed/9068580.

Nisker, J.A. "Chalcedonies." *Canadian Medical Association Journal* 164(1) (2001): 74–75.

Nisker, J. *Love and Injustice in Medicine: Annotated Narrative Ethics Explorations.* Toronto: Iguana Books, 2022.

Chapter IV—Beneath the BMW's Wheels

Hesse, H. *Beneath the Wheel.* New York: Farrar, Straus and Giroux, 1968.

Nisker, J. "Homeless Beneath a BMW's Wheels." *Canadian Medical Association Journal,* 192(28) (2020): E815–E816.

Troper, H., and E. Abella. *None Is Too Many: Canada and the Jews of Europe, 1933–1948.* Toronto: Lester & Orpen Dennys, 1982.

Trudeau, P. "Canada Must Be a Just Society." CBC Digital Archives. Video, September 9, 1968, 2:20. http://www.cbc.ca/player/play/1797431608.

Chapter V—COVID Injustice Before I Heard the Word "COVID"

Dolgin, E. "Omicron Thwarts Some of the World's Most-Used COVID Vaccines." *Nature* 601(7893) (2022), 311. https://doi.org/10.1038/d41586-022-00079-6.

Khandia, R., S. Singhal, T. Alqahtani, M.A. Kamal, N.A. El-Shall, F. Nainu, P.A. Desingu, and K. Dhama. "Emergence of SARS-CoV-2 Omicron (B.1.1.529) Variant, Salient Features, High Global Health Concerns and Strategies to Counter It amid Ongoing COVID-19 Pandemic." *Environ Res* (2022). doi: 10.1016/j.envres.2022.112816. Epub ahead of print. PMID: 35093310; PMCID: PMC8798788.

Kim, H. "Nearly 10% of North Korea's Population Sick amid COVID Outbreak." CBC News, May 19, 2022. https://www.cbc.ca/news/world/north-korea-covid-cases-outbreak-1.6460337.

Kolnes, N.H., S.N. Eikeland, T.A. Ersdal, and G.S. Braut. "Estimating the Consequences of a COVID-19 Super Spreader: A Stochastic Model of a Night on the Town." *Scandinavian Journal of Public Health* 50(1) (2022): 111–16. https://doi.org/10.1177/14034948211031400.

Li, X.P., S. Ullah, H. Zahir, A. Alshehri, M.B. Riaz, and B.A. Alwan. "Modeling the Dynamics of Coronavirus with Super-Spreader Class: A Fractal-Fractional Approach." *Results in Physics* 34 (2022): 105179. https://doi.org/10.1016/j.rinp.2022.105179.

Marchand, L. "Passengers on Sunwing Party Plane Could Face Jail Time, Thousands in Fines." CBC News (January 5, 2022). https://www.cbc.ca/news/canada/montreal/sunwing-cancun-flight-1.6304854.

Nisker, J. *Love and Injustice in Medicine: Annotated Narrative Ethics Explorations*. Toronto: Iguana Books, 2022.

Wang, N. *In the Same Breath*. HBO Original Documentary, 2021.

World Health Organization. "WHO-Convened Global Study of Origins of SARS-CoV-2: China Part [Internet]." World Health Organization (January 14–February 10, 2021). https://www.who.int/publications/i/item/who-convened-global-study-of-origins-of-sars-cov-2-china-part.

Zeitchik, S. "A Scathing New Documentary from HBO Alleges a Chinese Coverup on the Coronavirus." *Washington Post*, January 28, 2021. https://www.washingtonpost.com/business/2021/01/28/china-hbo-covid-film/.

Chapter VI—COVID Aggression Condemns a Muslim Family Near Our Medical School

Dolynny, T. "Second Person Wanted in Connection with Western Student's Death." CBC News, September 17, 2021. https://www.cbc.ca/news/canada/london/second-person-wanted-in-connection-with-western-student-s-death-1.6180684.

Dubinski, K. "Arrests Made after 4 Western Students Reported Sexual Assaults in Past Week, University Official Says." CBC News, September 13, 2021. https://www.cbc.ca/news/canada/london/western-campus-sexual-violence-reports-1.6173443.

Chapter VII—Ruth

Nisker, J. "Calcedonies: Critical Reflections on Writing Plays to Engage Citizens in Health and Social Policy Development." *Reflective Practice* 11(4) (2010): 417–32.

Nisker, J. "Calcedonies." In *Health Humanities Reader*, edited by T. Jones, D. Wear, and L.D. Friedman, Chapter 42. New Brunswick, NJ: Rutgers University Press, 2014.

Nisker J. "Chalcedonies." In *From the Other Side of the Fence: Stories from Health Care Professionals*, edited by J. Nisker, 172–76. Halifax: Pottersfield Press, 2008.

Nisker, J. *From Calcedonies to Orchids: Plays Promoting Humanity in Health Policy*. Toronto: Iguana Books, 2012.

Nisker, J. *Love and Injustice in Medicine: Annotated Narrative Ethics Explorations*. Toronto: Iguana Books, 2022.

Nisker, J. *Patiently Waiting For...* Toronto: Iguana Books, 2015.

Nisker, J.A. "The Yellow Brick Road of Medical Education." *Canadian Medical Association Journal,* *156*(5) (1997): 689–91. https://www.ncbi.nlm.nih.gov/pubmed/9068580.

Nisker, J.A. "Chalcedonies." *Canadian Medical Association Journal* 164(1) (2001): 74–75.

Chapter VIII—Antivaxxer Xenophobic COVID Violence

"COVID-19 Protesters Demonstrate across Canada in Support of Truck Convoy in Ottawa." CBC News, January 29, 2022. https://www.cbc.ca/news/canada/canada-protests-truck-convy-1.6332680.

"Frustration Mounts as Blockade Snarling Access to U.S. Border Continues at Alberta Port of Entry." CBC News, January 31, 2022. https://www.cbc.ca/news/canada/calgary/blockade-coutts-alberta-trucker-covid-convoy-1.6333957.

"Protesters Continue to Blockade Major Canada–U.S. Border Crossing in Manitoba." CBC News, February 12, 2022. https://www.cbc.ca/news/canada/manitoba/protest-canada-us-border-blockade-manitoba-1.6349659.

"The Convoy Crisis in Ottawa: A Timeline of Key Events." CBC News, February 17, 2022. https://www.cbc.ca/news/canada/ottawa/timeline-of-convoy-protest-in-ottawa-1.6351432.

Andrews, B., and A. Anand. "After Weekend of Protests, Ottawa Residents Are Feeling the Effects." CBC News, January 31, 2022. https://www.cbc.ca/news/canada/ottawa/convoy-workers-two-days-later-1.6333017.

Brown, H.K., S. Saha, T. Chan, A.M. Cheung, M. Fralick, M. Ghassemi, M. Herridge, et al. "Outcomes in Patients with and without Disability Admitted to Hospital with COVID-19: A Retrospective Cohort Study." *Canadian Medical Association Journal* 194(4) (2022): E112–E121. https://doi.org/10.1503/cmaj.211277.

Daigle, T. "In This Ontario Hospital, It's Mostly the Unvaccinated Who Are Overwhelming the ICU." CBC News, January 15, 2022. https://www.cbc.ca/news/health/sarnia-bluewater-health-hospital-covid-patients-1.6315681.

Dwyer, J. "Pandemic individualism." *Impact Ethics Blog*, February 3, 2022. https://impactethics.ca/2022/02/03/pandemic-individualism/.

Favaro, A., and A. Jones. "Inside an ICU Where 70 Per Cent of COVID-19 Patients Are Unvaccinated." CTV News, January 12, 2022. https://www.ctvnews.ca/health/coronavirus/inside-an-icu-where-70-per-cent-of-covid-19-patients-are-unvaccinated-1.5738198.

Fraser, K. "Ambassador Bridge Reopens with Heavy Police Presence Around Former Windsor, Ont., Protest Site." CBC News, February 14, 2022. https://www.cbc.ca/news/canada/windsor/ambassador-bridge-reopens-monday-1.6350729.

Green, M.J., P. Croskerry, and R. Rieck. "Annals Graphic Medicine—Bed Blocker." *Annals of Internal Medicine* 172(11) (2020): W142–W148. https://doi.org/10.7326/G20-0001.

Habib, M. "Occupy Canada Rallies Spread in Economic 'Awakening'." CBC News, October 13, 2011. https://www.cbc.ca/news/canada/occupy-canada-rallies-spread-in-economic-awakening-1.1031793.

Kannan, S., P. Shaik Syed Ali, and A. Sheeza. "Omicron (B.1.1.529)—Variant of Concern—Molecular Profile and Epidemiology: A Mini Review." *European Review for Medical and Pharmacological Sciences* 25(24) (2021): 8019–22. https://doi.org/10.26355/eurrev_202112_27653.

Khandia, R., S. Singhal, T. Alqahtani, M.A. Kamal, N.A. El-Shall, F. Nainu, P.A. Desingu, and K. Dhama. "Emergence of SARS-CoV-2 Omicron (B.1.1.529) Variant, Salient Features, High Global Health Concerns and Strategies to Counter It amid Ongoing COVID-19 Pandemic." *Environ Res* 2022. doi: 10.1016/j.envres.2022.112816. Epub ahead of print. PMID: 35093310; PMCID: PMC8798788.

Kolnes, N.H., S.N. Eikeland, T.A. Ersdal, and G.S. Braut. "Estimating the Consequences of a COVID-19 Super Spreader: A Stochastic Model of a Night on the Town." *Scandinavian Journal of Public Health* 50(1) (2022): 111–16. https://doi.org/10.1177/14034948211031400.

Li, X.P., S. Ullah, H. Zahir, A. Alshehri, M.B. Riaz, and B.A. Alwan. "Modeling the Dynamics of Coronavirus with Super-Spreader Class: A Fractal-Fractional Approach." *Results in Physics* 34 (2022): 105179. https://doi.org/10.1016/j.rinp.2022.105179.

Lord, C. "Trucker Convoy: Trudeau Says Protest 'Becoming Illegal' as Demands for Action Grow." *Global News*, February 2, 2022. https://globalnews.ca/video/8587818/like-were-being-held-hostage-ottawa-residents-frustrated-as-truck-protesters-refuse-to-leave.

McGrail, K.M., R.G. Evans, M.L. Barer, S.B. Sheps, C. Hertzman, and A. Kazanjian. "The Quick and the Dead: 'Managing' Inpatient Care in British Columbia Hospitals, 1969–1995/96." *Health Services Research* 35(6) (2001): 1319–38.

Reston, M., and K. Liptak. "The Day America Realized How Dangerous Donald Trump Is." *CNN Politics*, January 9, 2021. https://www.cnn.com/2021/01/09/politics/donald-trump-dangerous-capitol-riot/index.html.

Steinbeck, J. *The Grapes of Wrath.* New York: The Viking Press-James Lloyd, 1939.

Styrborn, K., and M. Thorslund. "Delayed Discharge of Elderly Hospital Patients—A Study of Bed-Blockers in a Health Care District in Sweden." *Scandinavian Journal of Social Medicine* 21(4) (1993): 272–80. https://doi.org/10.1177/140349489302100407.

Tasker, J.P. "Thousands Opposed to COVID-19 Rules Converge on Parliament Hill." *CBC News*, January 29, 2022. https://www.cbc.ca/news/politics/truck-convoy-protest-some-key-players-1.6332312.

Chapter IX—She Lived with the Knowledge

Nisker, J. *From Calcedonies to Orchids: Plays Promoting Humanity in Health Policy.* Toronto: Iguana Books, 2012.

Chapter X—Victor

Nisker, J. *Love and Injustice in Medicine: Annotated Narrative Ethics Explorations*. Toronto: Iguana Books, 2022.

Chapter XII—Our Third COVID Summer

Elliot, T.S. "The Love Song of J. Alfred Prufrock." *Poetry: A Magazine of Verse*, 1915.